Why I Quit: Reflections on a Fitness Instructor Career

ARZU GOSNEY

DEDICATION

This book is dedicated to my wonderful husband
Greg Gosney,
And to my beautiful children
Melisa Sencer Gosney and Burak Gosney.

CONTENTS

ACKNOWLEDGMENTS

Tom Corson-Knowles; This guy is a genius. I have been following his books and podcasts for awhile now and love his straightforward approach and genuine desire to help other self publishing authors. I hope he knows that he is helping many that he doesn't even know/met. His podcasts that I am addicted to answered the questions that I wanted to ask at the right time, almost reading my mind. When I was feeling down, he gave me the inspiration to continue on and for that I am forever grateful and a follower for his legit business that is centered around helping others, Thank you Tom!

Tricia Petrinovich; I have met Tricia through one of my fitness training session that she hosted in her beautiful studio. I appreciated her opening her doors to me back than and we engaged in conversations about Tricia's fiction book since it was taking place in a country that I grew up in, Turkey! I remember the coffee date after my training, probably I was stinky and tired but tried to help her as much as possible at the same time. Tricia came back to my rescue after the initial electronic copy of my book. She helped me with editing and offered her amazing talent to me while keeping my voice throughout my book at the same. I am grateful to have met you and thank you so much Tricia!

Alan N Kim Patterson-Burkhardt; she is my partner in crime in my fitness journey. This memoir that covers for the most part of my trainer journey, this girl knows all my ups and downs of being a fitness instructor. We cried on each others shoulders and laughed hard together. She has been with me on my good days, and she has been with me on my bad and for that we are true best friends forever. Once a friend, always a friend, thank you Kim!

Greg Gosney; last but not least! This man is not only my soul mate but also my rock. He is my courageous fighter, he is my hardworking role model that I continue to learn so much from! He brings loving tears to my eyes every time I see him. He is the one, who saw the book in the early stages and knowing everything, he is the one who pushed me out of my comfort zone. When we were on our date night dinner, he is the one who told me "If you are going to write a book, you have to write it all. Why hide anything? Why would you not say anything about this and that and the elevator?" Oh, the elevator! He is the one who I discussed the "without further ado" vs "without further adieu" with! Greg is my better half, he is a true leader and an amazing dad and a husband. I love you Greg and thank you so much for brightening up my day with your presence, every day!

1 WHY I WROTE THIS BOOK

I have been a huge dance fitness enthusiast, investing all of my energy and passion into it - just like the other millions of instructors and students worldwide. If you are in the early stages of teaching or taking dance fitness classes, I understand your excitement. I understand how much you love your class and how you think it has changed your life and given you new meaning. I understand because I have been there. *I understand.* That is what the company thrives on. So much passion goes into dance fitness and the class experience, and your energy is contagious. Subsequently, this industry has grown enormously.

Over my six years of being a dance fitness instructor, it is safe to say that I have some experience under my belt. (In the equivalent time of a college career, I would have a Master's Degree!) That is not to say that I claim to know it all. Of course there is always more to learn! But I can say that in the end, instructing dance fitness classes had become a part of my *nature.* And turning my back on all of it was like severing a part of me. It required far more courage than I would have imagined.

Once you read this book, you may understand why I made this decision. Regardless of whether you agree with my choice, my goal is to give you, the reader, an idea of what goes on behind the scenes so that you might reconsider your actions and future aspirations with the perspective of this book.

Let me put it this way: There are two sides to every coin, but lying flat on a table, only one side is clearly visible. I have seen the other side that has been invisible to you so far. Not everyone gets to see it, because the other side requires getting into the industry at a different level. But if I can describe it for you and tell you what I saw and how it looks, you can formulate a picture in your mind. And then you can decide if it is a coin you want to keep. Or to decide how much you are willing to do to get it.

Even if you are not in the fitness industry this book can still provide value. You may be able to apply its perspective if you find yourself in a similar challenge of making a hard decision in your life. The lesson that there is often more under the surface or within the inner layers of an organization, entity or group is transferrable. This book might prompt you to dig deeper and acquire more information in order to make the decision that is right for you.

2 WHY YOU SHOULD READ THIS BOOK

If you are a fitness instructor, in the process of becoming an instructor, or are advancing your career within the fitness industry: This book is a must-read. I give you my own experiences, and the reflections of a fitness career from start to finish can hold tremendous value to any reader who is even remotely considering a career within the industry. I wish that I had access to such a resource when I first started my journey. It may not have swayed my decision (sometimes we insist on finding out for ourselves - no matter what!) but it would have been valuable to have filed away the experiences of someone else so that I could have recognized the warning signs earlier. And it might have provided much-needed guidance in making decisions along the way.

I will warn you, however: *This book can be viewed as controversial.* Remember my analogy of the coin? I am uncovering some things that only those who have gotten much deeper into the industry have seen. Some people don't want to know much about that side. They want to keep looking at the clearly visible part under the gleaming light that is, well, *shiny*! The part in the shadows close to the table can stay hidden. Others are more affiliated with the other side, the invisible part. And they don't want someone to describe their side to anyone else.

But my goal is simple - to make sure you do know that *there are two sides*, so that you can think about how much you want to know and see. You can decide for yourself if that other side will affect your own adventure in the industry.

Last but most importantly: Thank you for your purchase! And as you read, I only ask that you please keep an open mind.

3 INTRODUCTION

Being a fitness instructor has never been my main occupation. By day, I am a computer scientist. I know, right? Hardly what anyone would think for the alter ego of a dance fitness instructor! In reading the earlier pages, you already know I had endless passion for dance fitness. But can I also say - I *love* my technical job and working in management. How many people can say that? But it is true. I love my day job as a scientist, and I lead a technical group at a highly respected multi-billion dollar national research laboratory.

In addition, I am an entrepreneur, the mom in a blended family, and a wife. Of course, these other roles played a part in my fitness journey (and the need to balance everything) but this book will focus on my dance fitness instructor career and not the other side of my life. But you need to know about it and that instructing fitness classes was not my only "job." It helps put things in perspective.

You may also have guessed that I cannot identify the dance fitness company for whom I worked due to trademark concerns. So I will refer it as company "X" and the position I took with the company as an "XYZ" throughout the remainder of the book.

This book is organized into five "Acts":

Act 1: Describes my dance fitness background. (Again, I don't spend a lot of time talking about myself in general - you can read all you want about me on my Web site. Instead, I share this so you can find where your story resonates with mine depending on the stage you are in with your fitness journey.)

Act 2: Delves into the details of how I became an XYZ with company X.

Act 3: Is about my second year as an XYZ and what changes I was experiencing in that role.

Act 4: Discusses even more changes and challenges in my third and final year as an XYZ.

Act 5: Explores the reasons of my exit from it all.

Before you start reading, I want to make something clear. I will continue to support anybody in his or her journey to a healthy and fit lifestyle. And if a particular dance fitness program is what is getting them there, I will encourage it. I have expertise in taking *and* instructing dance fitness classes, and I am willing to share the information I have with anybody who wants to learn it. I believe in helping other people to become productive, improving their health and careers, and being happy and content with their lives.

I am also grateful for the opportunities I have had to impact the lives of dance fitness students, instructors and others. This experience gave me a new perspective on life and taught me about my own priorities and values. It opened numerous doors and provided opportunities that helped me start new businesses and grow. For all these reasons I will forever be grateful for the chance I had to teach dance fitness classes and for all the friendships that I made throughout the journey.

Now let's get started.

ACT I
MY BACKGROUND

4 HOW I BECAME AN INSTRUCTOR

It was the end of 2007. I was eight months pregnant and feeling big! I gained 50 pounds during each of my pregnancies. A future with a new baby in front of me, I was trying to find a gym to attend after the baby was born. It was going to be part of my new year's resolution (I know you can relate).

I came across a new, small, women's-only gym close to our house. One day after work, my husband and I stopped by to get a flyer. It is funny because up until that day I had never belonged to a gym or purchased a gym membership. Speaking with the owner (who could see I was very far along in a pregnancy), I explained that I would start the gym after having the baby. I told her we were just there to get a flyer. As she was trying to build clientele in her new business, she told me to go ahead and register and said she would start the monthly dues after the baby was born. In other words, I could use the gym at my leisure before the baby was born. Also, I would be able to cancel at any time. Having nothing to lose, I joined that day.

I was a bit nervous at first. I thought (being so noticeably pregnant) that everybody would be watching me if I were to take a class. So I started slow and easy, just using the treadmill. I used to jog in my bedroom on my own treadmill, but I wasn't used to exercising with people around me. I was delighted to find the women in the gym extremely nice and supportive. And who wouldn't be towards an eight month pregnant lady, right?

This was my second pregnancy, and I could tell my body was adjusting well to the exercise so I decided to take a group fitness class after all. These were held in the basement of the gym. I took various classes teaching different formats when I felt up to it. But I hadn't tried X. Yet. Not that I didn't want to - I just didn't know what it was! Eventually the owner told me that I should try it, describing it as a "fun dance fitness class." I had never taken a formal dance lesson before, but I liked dancing so why not?

From that first class I was hooked. I thought it was like the best class *ever*. I loved how it made me feel. Oh so happy! I was doing all the moves to the level my pregnant body would allow, loving every second of it and having so much fun. All the ladies were so friendly and for the first time, I started to have friends outside of my day job.

I actually participated in an X class on my due date (don't worry, I made it!), but was induced the next day. Can you believe I was back at the gym taking my fun X classes three weeks after my son was born? I almost had to re-learn the moves (who knows what having a baby does to your brain!) but I still was having so much fun with it. To me it was never about weight loss. I took the classes because I *loved* them so much. And it never crossed my mind that one day I would teach a fitness class. I was always the business and technology minded girl in class or at work.

Two months after giving birth to my son, I received a call from a former roommate who was working in Chicago. She informed me she had accepted yet-another-job in England so she was going to be leaving the States. She asked if I would like to see her before she left. Talking it over with my husband, we decided that it might be a good idea for me to have a break for a couple of days. My parents were staying with us to help out with the baby, and (most importantly) I had plenty of milk pumped - !

Still trying to convince myself of the value of the trip, I checked out the X website and saw that there was an instructor training scheduled during the dates we were talking about meeting. At the time, there were not many instructor trainings in Washington State, where I was living at the time. So this added another reason to go. I suggested to my friend that we take the X training together, something that might be fun to do. She agreed. Even after registering for the training I was not planning to teach classes. I just saw it as something I was intrigued by and wanted to learn more about.

On the very day I was supposed to fly to Chicago for my training, the owner of the women-only gym I had joined held her grand opening. (She had delayed it in order to have it outdoors.) The gym's X instructor was doing a demo as part of the event and had asked for students to help her out during her part. I was one of the volunteers. So, my husband, parents and kids came to see me do what I had been telling them so much about and what I had just registered to attend training for. Being perhaps a *bit* biased, my husband told me how impressed he was with how well I knew and performed the dance moves. He mentioned, after seeing the grand opening demonstration, that the training in Chicago was going to be a good experience no matter what happened following my return from visiting my friend. (As you might have guessed, my husband is a great guy. But that is a subject for a different book...)

I will never forget the training in Chicago! It was a long day with numerous trips to the ladies room (I was pumping milk for the baby). I was exhausted by the end of the training but had so much fun! I saw a very different side of the program, including some intense X that I had never seen in prior classes up to that time.

My friend, who had no idea about exercise or dance fitness, was clueless as to what she was doing. I caught the trainer eyeing her a few times but, since there were no requirements to become an X instructor other than being present during the training and doing what they told you to the best of your ability, by the end of the day we were both granted the X fitness instructor title. This wasn't a big deal for my friend, but for me it was enormous! I was exhausted, but full of joy.

And yet... even though my friend and I both received the license to teach X fitness classes and I was excited, I still thought this was something I was supposed to keep it to myself. How little did I know!

5 TEACHING CLASSES, WHAT, ME?!?!?

The week after returning from the training, the owner of the gym told me that the X instructor had hurt her ankle and that her doctor advised her to stop teaching. She knew I had just obtained my instructor license and, at the time, there were not many people in town licensed to teach X classes. She asked if I could start teaching. The idea of teaching a fitness class was foreign, and I felt uncomfortable about it. Still, I liked a good challenge and knew I had a passion for teaching so I agreed to do it.

I had one week to get ready for the class. One week! I remember going to the gym every day after the baby was asleep. Boy did I work hard to get ready. In fact, the day of my first class my husband had to pop the blisters that had formed on the soles of my feet. It was unbearable to walk, let alone dance!

I remember my first class as if it were today. And let me just say - it wasn't the best. I remember all the negative thoughts that were going through my mind: "What am I doing?" and "I'm not cut out for this!" and "I've never taught a fitness class before! Am I crazy?"

I struggled mentally and worried that my negative thoughts would be recognizable to the others I was teaching and therefore impact the class. To my relief and surprise the ladies who attended approached me after class and stated how much fun they had and encouraged me that the class was great. Instead of believing them, however, I thought they were just being polite and supportive while surely inside they shared the same thoughts as me. Although I wrestled with quitting, somehow the positive feedback helped me decide that I needed to give myself a chance to get better at this type of a teaching experience. And I felt I was in a safe place.

The second class was like night-and-day compared to my first. Who knew it could turn around so quickly? That follow-up experience gave me the biggest boost in my decision to continue. In fact, I never looked back from that point. Of course, I could talk about all the lessons learned and the hard work that I put into my first year as a dance fitness instructor but that would, again, take the length of another book!

6 FURTHERING EDUCATION

Later in 2008, I completed the necessary training to receive an additional license to teach at another level within company X. It proved even more of a learning experience, and I started to get involved with the growing X community in our town and even started teaching at other gyms and dance studios.

In 2009, I obtained my first accredited fitness certification from the "Aerobics and Fitness Association of America" (AFAA) for "group exercise." Later, I added certifications as "personal trainer" and in tele-fitness. I believe in education and wanted to make my classes better. It didn't sit well with me that I could continue to teach classes by attending a single day of training per the X format and structure. I wanted to learn more about the fitness industry so that I not only provided fun and engaging dance fitness classes, but so I would be better trained in safe (and unsafe) moves, injury prevention, healthy bodies, and more. I wanted to be an educated instructor both for my current students as well as for my growing clientele. And I wanted them to be able to come to me with questions and concerns in relation to any type of fitness, health, nutrition, or even dance-related topics.

In addition to obtaining my certifications, I was also reading and researching information related to these topics. I was still enjoying myself immensely and was having much success at this point in time. So much so that my husband and I decided to go to the instructor conference in Orlando in 2010 (and have a family vacation at the same time).

The instructor conference was a great way to network and was overall an exciting experience. If you are in the fitness industry, I highly recommend attending a conference if you are able to. If nothing else, it is just a boost to be surrounded by thousands of like-minded people. You receive inspiration and are able to speak the same language, share the same passion, exchange ideas, and help each other. I was meeting new people from all over, as well as the fitness celebrities that I was watching on the infomercials and DVDs. In fact, all was going well until a little incident in the elevator.

My husband and I were in the hotel, traveling back to our room. Somehow our elevator passed our floor and went all the way up to the top floor of the hotel. (And no, it was not a free upgrade!) When the door opened, the very head and face of the fitness company I represented stepped into the elevator accompanied by his personal assistant! We had to have looked like deer in headlights.

My husband whispered to me, "Isn't that *him*?"

I said "Yes!" and then subsequently asked for a picture with him while heading back down in the elevator. There I was in full X gear, a huge enthusiast and a hardworking representative of the company. I had traveled literally across the country to be able to attend this conference for the company that this very man co-founded.

He said, "Sure."

My husband whipped out his phone and attempted to take the picture of the two of us together. But somehow, he missed the button. There was no picture on the phone! We then asked if he would mind if we tried again. The response was a bit shocking - the man uttered an unexpected reaction of frustration that bordered on anger! We went ahead and tried one more time but something went wrong again, and we still didn't have a picture. As you can imagine, we were not going to ask a third time.

My husband was extremely bothered, even angry, by the co-founder's unprofessional, impatient and rude reaction to us. I was able to calm him down by explaining that perhaps he was having a bad day or had something else on his mind? I told him that we just needed to let it go. We did, but from my husband's perspective, this was the very person I was supporting through my hours of time, my investment of money and all of my efforts to grow my X business. And the bottom line is that my husband would defend me in the same way if he saw me being treated badly by *anyone*...celebrity or not.

As young as our kids were at the time, my husband had done most of the babysitting during the conference. The event lasted three days, but I was able to spend the rest of the time with them and we all enjoyed our family vacation. Overall I was really happy with my first instructor conference experience and loved it. In fact, I had gotten two additional X format licenses during the trip, furthering my education even more, and we caught up with family time. All was good.

Early in 2011, I applied for another position within company X. In this new role I sought, I would be the person teaching the trainings; the one helping others to get their license to become instructors. However, I was not selected. Feeling a bit of a setback, I decided to just keep doing what I had been doing – finding love and joy in teaching classes.

Then, in mid-2011, company X issued a call for a new position, something they called an XYZ. This new program was launched due to the company's surging growth of its instructor network. An XYZ would focus primarily on teaching choreography. Instead of an all-day training, a class would be a targeted session that lasted a few hours and would be at a reduced cost compared to the all-day trainings. The goal was to create a safe environment for instructors to share ideas, network, receive inspiration, and learn choreography with the lead of an experienced instructor.

I remember the backlash from some of the instructors, who had no idea what the program was about, and all the discussions questioning the value of the program when instructors could learn dance choreography from YouTube, social media, other dance videos, DVDs, and more. On the other hand, I really liked the idea from the outset and thought the backlash was due to the growing competition that was forming due to the expanding instructor network. In other words, I attributed the controversy to the growing pains that any business goes through.

Although there was validity to some of the discussions, I had faith in the company and the vision that was set. With my passion for the program, my teaching skills, and the sum of my knowledge and experience so far, I thought I would be a good candidate for this position. Not only would it continue to further my skills and knowledge, but there was an additional earning potential with this new program as well.

I reviewed my journey thus far. I had 2 years of teaching dance fitness classes. It had started in the basement of a small women's only gym, but had evolved into helping other gyms around town and subbing as needed, even venturing out on my own to rent dance studios. I had volunteered at charity and fundraising events, hosted classes at corporate venues and other community events. I was getting involved in many different types of "gigs!"

There were weeks that I taught as many as 13 classes, in addition to another special event, fundraiser or demo that I had committed to. Although it was overwhelming, I had created a lot of buzz with hard work and passion. Some of these classes and events were for-profit, and I made good income at the dance studios I had rented. Other classes and events were not-for-profit, engaged in just to benefit an organization or charity. At times, events I was volunteering for were so successful that people were grateful and generous, acknowledging my time and effort by writing me checks, which I would then split with the applicable non-profit organization.

The point was that I was putting a lot of time and energy into the teaching side of the business and it was paying off. In fact, I was so dialed-in that at times all I had to do to get ready for a class, demo or event was to just listen to the music in my car and focus while traveling to or from work. All the hard work during my first year was yielding results! I was super quick at picking up new choreography, and extremely efficient at using the technology, tools, and software that made my life easier and helped me succeed during that time frame.

I might also mention that during this same period, I had other professional projects brewing. I had completed most of the schoolwork for my doctorate degree in computer science, and I knuckled under and finished the research project to receive my PhD during this time as well. In other words, dance fitness was becoming a part of me, having (literally) *worked* its way into my nature. My early investment was making it come easier to me and was resulting in big rewards, at times monetarily, although it was not just about the earning potential. As you can imagine, dance fitness was a needed stress relief from my day job and educational pursuits.

I also loved the people-aspect of teaching dance fitness. I loved seeing the smiling faces and helping others. And I wanted to set the example that you could fit health and fitness into your daily schedule no matter how "busy" you are.

Considering everything in perspective at the time, I

believed applying for the new XYZ position was a great opportunity for me in my dance fitness instructor career. I believed I was qualified and needed to give it a try because of how far and fast I had seen company X grow.

You see, the buzz had spread rapidly and company X's advertising efforts were helping every instructor in the field, including me. But the increased demand for X meant the need for more instructors. Consequently, instructor training sessions were held all over the place and, with people becoming instructors by just attending a day of training with no additional requirements, new instructors were launching classes at a rapid rate. After two years, the market was now getting a bit saturated. And yet it seemed that as the earning potential was slowing down (due to more and more offered classes), that even *more* instructors were coming on board.

Competition is a good thing. An increase in local instructors means you need to stay on your "A" game to rise to the top. For me, I saw exploring this new opportunity as an XYZ as a way for me to be a leader of X in my community. Since the challenge and achievement of obtaining my PhD was behind me, I believed I was ready to take this on.

I gingerly sent in my videos and submission package, a little nervous due to my prior denied application from company X. I heard (but have no way to substantiate) that there were over 4000 first round applications and that they selected 89 of those applicants to be the first group of XYZ's. Imagine my surprise when I was one who was selected! Feeling elated, I booked my flight and made our family vacation reservations for the second year in a row to the instructor conference. This time, I had to arrive a day early to take a training scheduled before the convention would start. I was so stoked!

The XYZ training was a one day session that lasted five to six hours. We were told the purpose of the program and then were trained on the basic outline for the sessions we would teach when we got back home. Throughout the day, we received inspiration by well-intentioned and passionate people like us who already had obtained other contractor positions within the company.

One of the things explained to us was that company X was changing their software platform and that a new portal would be available within a month for us to start scheduling our sessions. Other than that, it would be up to us to improve this program. All was great so far!

Then, towards the end of the session, the head of the company (remember the elevator story?) made his appearance and put in a few inspirational words, gave tips from his experience and introduced us to the new teenage girls that he had discovered off of YouTube. They then showed us the new songs they had been working on for the convention DVDs. Huh?

You see, within that very training, YouTube had been explained to us as forbidden by the company. The reasoning made sense and was all related to protecting the brand as well as the choreography of the people who put hours into it. And here was a presentation of new talent discovered on the same forbidden platform by the head of the company! Don't get me wrong. The girls were sweethearts, humble, great dancers, and gorgeous, but nevertheless the message sent towards the XYZ's and other educators that were present at the training was a bit confusing and hypocritical.

Despite this hypocrisy, I told myself that I just needed to stay focused on my own goals and how I could grow through this experience and in this new position. I was committed to being true to myself and to the people who were supporting me back at my small hometown. I decided that I still needed to hold on to the torch and lead the way.

Oh, and one last thing. At the end of the training, every XYZ was able to take their picture with the man who headed up the company! So on what was essentially my third try (and a year later), I finally got my picture with the man from the elevator....

ACT II
THE FIRST YEAR, ROUGH START

7 LATE START

Coming back from the training and "family vacation," I was tired and felt I needed a vacation-after-the-vacation. But I was excited to get started with the new program just like all the other new official XYZ's and decided to jump right in. It turns out that was not to happen. The new portal, announced at our training as ready one month out, was delayed. Now we were told that the XYZ software portal would not be available for about three months. This meant nobody was able to set up schedules for the new XYZ program.

The new XYZ's were feeling a bit frustrated, but as a computer scientist I understood the pains of launching a new software portal on a new platform and all the project scope issues that could creep in and create delays. I dealt with that at my day job on a daily basis. However, I didn't want to sit around and wait!

We were told at the training that the portal would not receive payments for the sessions we would schedule, so we were to collect money for the registrations with other means on our own. Therefore, I got to work. I put in a substantial amount of my own money and time into building my own website with all the elements required to launch this program. It required setting up all of the tools required for this program to take off. I even hired my best friend as my assistant to help me with the registrations and marketing of my training sessions. Finally, the program launched and I was READY.

8 INITIAL REQUIREMENTS

When the XYZ program first launched, we were given a lot of flexibility. Essentially, a basic structure for the program had been drawn up for us, but it would be up to us to make it the most valuable for the instructors we were to provide our service for. As a former adjunct faculty at a college, I felt confident in my abilities to structure a class or training, so I created my own lesson plan.

The first step was to find a place to host our session. My assistant and I spent *hours* calling facilities and trying to convince them to host us. Remember, this was something "new" and not everyone was open to it. I remember it being a lot of hard work, just securing the location. But we eventually met with success.

Some of the cities and areas we visited had very few X instructors. When there, our intention was to "spread the love," knowing full well that there would not be many people present. We would then be excited when we booked a session in an area that we knew had an abundance of X instructors. Imagine our disappointment when we would still have low attendance! There were two factors seemingly at play. First, there were growing pains for this new program. Nobody knew who we were and what this program was about. Second, we learned that some instructors were content just paying monthly dues to the company to get the DVDs. They weren't interested in the networking and live session format we brought to them. Even some of the instructors who were working at the very gyms where we were scheduled for the trainings were refusing to attend the sessions. We did encounter some open-minded and supportive instructors (both new and very experienced instructors) who attended the sessions, were thankful for our visit and provided great feedback. But these supportive folks were in the minority.

Another difficulty we encountered was there was not always a good way of reaching out to the instructors who *would* love to be at the sessions. I remember our efforts involving working with established trainers, other XYZs, and instructors in these areas - inviting them to my sessions.

During my sessions, I worked hard to bond with every attendee, and I genuinely wanted to help each and every person. I was assisting the experienced instructors to get to the next level in their career; I was trying to help the new instructors with the most crucial tips that they needed to know early on in their careers. I was not only putting all my choreography efforts and sweat during these sessions and master classes - I was also spreading the program like wild fire.

In the midst of preparing for my current sessions, I was working on how to grow the program. I would use online tools as well as other forms of invitation for registrations to invite other trainers of the X program to my sessions. I wanted other XYZ's to come to my sessions to exchange ideas. In my first year, after attending my sessions, some of the XYZ's changed the format of their sessions.

My assistant would also provide honest feedback after each session. I processed the feedback I was hearing, seeing, feeling and then incorporate it to continue to improve my own format. I would share my experience as to what was and was not working with other XYZ's because I knew if we were all successful it was good for attendees, for the company, as well as for the XYZ program overall. I was continuously sharing and communicating all aspects of my fitness career, and I was implementing the new ideas I was hearing on the forums and receiving from other excellent and passionate XYZ's whose hearts and minds were in the same place. (I still have so many instructors from my sessions who are now my good friends on social media. Even though we are miles apart, we still keep in touch. They are all very special people in my life.)

I was having success and enjoying my role as an XYZ. At this time, there were no "minimum session requirements" set by the company, and I was scheduling sessions at my own pace. I didn't feel extraneous pressure to fit in a certain number of trainings each year, so I was able to make this career work with my already full-time schedule and family life.

Towards the end of the first year as an XYZ, the company did convey a standard of wanting us to hold at least six sessions every year. As this was in line with what I was currently doing anyway, I felt this was achievable. Things seemed to be going well.

9 LACK OF TOOLS AND SUPPORT

Although the quality and quantity of my sessions were extremely successful, XYZ's in general were dealing with a lack of company-provided support and tools, both for the registration of our sessions and in the area of communication. In other words, there were no reliable tools or processes in place to enable us to contact the instructors around the areas that we were holding our sessions. This was very troublesome. I would create a message to the instructors for whom I had contact information, and my assistant would send out individual messages to anyone who lived close to the area, notifying them that we were holding the session(s). All the while, we knew that through the company website, my message may or may not reach the instructor, due to both spam filters and troublesome website glitches. This happened constantly, even though we were using the method introduced to us in our initial XYZ training. What bothered me most was that I felt like I was bugging everybody, but unfortunately there was just no another way. Some instructors were thanking us for letting them know but others were just plain irritated.

So, in our efforts to try to reach the instructors without

spamming them, many of the XYZ's started to utilize social media, primarily Facebook at the time, to notify the instructors that we were coming to their areas. My assistant and I started to spend hours "socializing" online, primarily on Facebook and later on Twitter. Of course, not every instructor was on Facebook and this was a slow process. But considering the lack of a centralized tool, this was just another way we attempted to reach out to our market.

Little did we know that in the company's eyes, what we viewed as a solution was, to them, a problem. The XYZ's had marketed so heavily on social media that company X noticed the trend, and we were told that we could no longer use social media to market our sessions. This came with a lot of frustration and backlash, this time from the XYZ's. How were we supposed to get the word out? Eventually our feedback made the company bring some exceptions to the rule as there was just no other way to reach out to whoever wanted or needed the trainings that we were scheduling.

Despite all of our marketing efforts, despite the high quality of sessions we provided, and despite the positive feedback from those who attended our trainings, the numbers at our initial sessions were much lower than I expected them to be. Yes, this was a new program and seemingly had to spread best by word-of-mouth, but there was a huge target market that was growing all the time. I had a few sold out sessions but they were very few, and very far in between.

10 GIVING MY ALL

As much time, money, mental and physical effort I had invested into my XYZ business the first year, I still had hopes that this program would take off. I believed in the value and had trust in my skills. Although I was giving my all, the return on investment was very low in comparison to all the time my assistant and I were spending on the launch. However, I weighed it out and still loved what I was doing. Not only was there a lot of personal satisfaction, but the fact that I was able to help anybody with an interest in an instructor career was well-aligned with my passion for teaching. And so I carried on.

ACT III
THE SECOND YEAR, SCRUTINY

11 PROGRAM WITH CHANGING RULES

Towards the end of my first year as an XYZ, we received a very direct email from the head office informing us of some important changes in the XYZ program requirements. The office decided to change the minimum session requirement. In fact, they doubled it! Instead of six sessions per year, we were required to hold a whopping 12! It seemed to be a sign that they wanted full-time contractors who called being an XYZ their main job, because how could someone with another "day job" manage it all?

In addition to the change to a minimum of 12 sessions per year, however, there was something else. There was going to be a second round of eliminations within the group of previously selected XYZ's. In order to decide who would stay, they asked for a full video recording from one of our training sessions. Then, based on what they saw and after a thorough evaluation of the feedback they had received from attendees out of our past sessions, they would make their decision.

12 SECOND ROUND ELIMINATIONS

I really had to think long and hard about this requirement change and come up with a "Go" or "No go" decision. I knew that I had to eliminate something if I was to continue. There was just no other way to fit 12 sessions into my already-full schedule. I had a heart-to-heart discussion with my husband. He felt that I had the time-management skills, experience and ability to quickly prepare for sessions and that I *could* meet this requirement. But, we both agreed, the question was: Should I?

While some might have resented the video submission requirement, it actually intrigued me. At that point in my career, I needed some affirmation. As XYZ's, we never received responses to our comments to the head office about our sessions. I personally never received a response to my emails or program improvement ideas. In addition, although we were specifically told to emphasize and encourage the instructors who attended our sessions to fill out session evaluations and surveys, we did not receive responses in regards to our own evaluations and comments. The results and reports of session attendee surveys as a whole were kept private and were never shared with us. To this day, I don't understand the reason why. But I thought at the time that this would be a way for me to know if I was getting the feedback I hoped for and that they approved of my sessions.

I also thought these adjustments to the program would spur the head office to finally come up with improvements to the program at their level. In other words, I hoped the revamp would eliminate the lack of tools and support that was impacting our marketing efforts and hampering communication. The changes they were making, including the second round of video eliminations, actually gave me a leap of faith that the office was also going to become serious about this program, listen to the feedback, and finally improve the communication and support we were desperately needing.

Quickly, I booked a session and recorded it from beginning to end, created a DVD and sent it to the front office per the requirement and by the due date. When the word came back that I was selected as an XYZ who would continue, I was excited! It was the affirmation I had hoped for. On the other hand, some of the XYZ's who were eliminated came as a complete shock to me. Many had seemed to book so many sessions, and I was surprised that they were gone while I was selected to continue.

So now I was off for my third year as an XYZ, humbled by the assurance from the company that my sessions were of high quality, but also well-aware that there was a new set of rules. This time, I was an experienced XYZ, and I had to meet a lot of expectations.

ACT IV
THE THIRD YEAR, SO LONG

13 FRANTIC SCHEDULE

After signing my new, extended contract, and shortly after getting a company email promising a brighter future for the program, I started scheduling more XYZ sessions than ever before – certainly more than I was used to! As a result, I was traveling more and incurring the costs associated with traveling, including accommodation costs and extended hours. An analysis of the sessions showed I was hardly breaking even! It wasn't that I wasn't making money, but I also knew that if you really looked at it including *all* of the costs (time spent networking, attending other events, traveling and lodging, travel expenses attending conferences, printing materials, etc.) it was a meager living at best. Of course, for someone without a day job or other responsibilities like I have, some of those costs might be considered routine. And with more time, the person who did this full-time could provide more focus and probably find additional ways to increase his or her income with innovative ideas, hard work, luck and patience. But it wasn't that way for me.

I had to decide if this was okay with me. Were the earnings enough? Eventually, I accepted it because I saw this as "my fun job," something that I did out of my passion for it. So I determined that my third year goal as an XYZ was less financial and more to meet the requirements (12 sessions per year) and wait to see the long-promised changes to the program finally be implemented by the home office. Surely the tools would have an impact on an XYZ's financial picture?

Besides the financial issue, there were costs to my family life. Initially, when traveling, I tried to take my family with me so we could have "mini-vacations". But two things happened: it would cost even that much more (especially when needing to eat out), plus I didn't like the feeling of leaving my husband and kids to go to the training while supposedly on a "mini-vacation" *with* my family. In fact, with the mad schedule we were on, I remember a time when I had two sessions scheduled in two different locations in the same day. I had to change in a Starbucks© bathroom in between and felt exhausted by the end of the day with no energy to even enjoy the rest of the day with my family! And I remember feeling sad because of it.

As a side note, I don't intend for this to discourage or condemn anyone who currently has family (and a day job) while pursuing a trainer career in the fitness industry. Your circumstances may be different and you and your family may have found a way to make it work for you. These were the the struggles *I* encountered, and maybe some who have family do relate and find themselves going through the same feelings. It may or may not be the determining factor (or even *a* factor) of whether to keep a dance fitness trainer job. The truth is that no matter how much we love what we do, we all go through different emotions. Sometimes we decide to pursue or to *not* pursue outside careers to provide for our families, and I respect both of those decisions.

About three months into this third year, a new requirement was put on us. This time, it had to do with the structure of our sessions. It needed to change to a unified format and required us to break the music into different parts, which meant editing the songs. I was fortunate in that I was already proficient with software applications; it was something different to try, and I was open to new ideas. Nevertheless, it started to take longer to prepare for sessions.

When I reached the halfway point of this third year, I had to evaluate. There were six months of frantic XYZ life behind me with zero improvements supporting the XYZs that had been promised from the front office. At this point, unfortunately, I started to become resentful.

14 THE MOVE

In mid-2013, six months into my third year as an XYZ (with a frantic and exhausting schedule), we were informed of an opportunity that would advance my husband's career. The catch was that the advancement required a move to a different state. We analyzed the pros and cons over and over again, and we decided that we had to take this opportunity, otherwise my husband's position at his current job was going to become stale. This was not an easy decision by any means. It meant leaving the area where our kids had roots and friends, our million dollar properties, my businesses and business contacts, our friends and hobbies, and had a huge potential impact on my day job. But we took a huge leap of faith for the sake of our blended family and accepted the job.

We traded our 5200 square foot home for a 500 square foot hotel room, for two months at least. Not only were we in a brand new state, but in addition, we became the custodial parents of my stepson who made the move with us. I went to a teleworking schedule for my day job, enrolled our three children into new schools and supported my husband in his new high-level position within the company. We also spent time looking at new houses and finally bought our current residence - our third home together. Though all of this was, of course, challenging, it was actually a blessing in disguise and an experience that brought our family closer than ever before. Every day things were happening that provided reassurance that we had made the right decision and that the move was "meant to be". Everything was turning out to be better than expected. I already knew that my husband and I were a great team, but this experience reassured me that we could overcome any challenge that was thrown our way.

Having to take time off from my frantic schedule, this experience also gave me a new meaning and perspective, forcing me to readjust my priorities, simplify my life, and let go of the things that were not adding value to "my" goals, "my" family situation and where I wanted to be 5 or 10 years from now. I felt liberated.

15 THE RESIGNATION LETTER

The caption above says it all. This new season in my life made my decision clear. I wrote a short, to-the-point resignation letter from my XYZ position, and it was easier to do than I thought. I didn't sweat over it as I knew this was the right decision for me. What was completely ironic is that this was the only time I got an immediate reply from the head office! They wished me good luck and assumed or implied that my decision was due to the fact that I couldn't meet the requirements (which I never mentioned in the resignation letter). See the email thread below:

On Mon, Jan 6, 2014 at 2:19 PM, Arzu Gosney <arzu.gosney@gmail.com> wrote:

Dear XYZ Committee,

I would like to inform you that I am resigning from my position as an XYZ for X effective January 6th, 2014. I thank you so much for giving me the opportunity to be able to help other instructors grow in their careers and help them become better instructors by conducting XYZ sessions during the last three years. I truly enjoyed working as a XYZ.

If I can be of any help during this transition or for future reference, please let me know,

Sincerely,

Arzu Gosney.

Dear Arzu,

While we are sad that you cannot commit to the new requirements and can no longer continue as an XYZ, we truly understand and respect your decision.

We thank you for the amount of time, effort, and commitment you have given to your sessions, participants, and the XYZ Program. The program has been defined by the hard work and effort of every XYZ and you will always be an important member of the instructor community.

We know you will continue changing lives with your passion for the X program and we wish you the very best in all your ventures.

Warm regards,

XYZ Committee

Getting over the XYZ position resignation quickly, the next step was resigning from being an instructor. I won't lie to you - this process was a bit harder for my heart, but I still thought that it was the right decision. So, I logged on to the instructor portal and clicked on the "cancel my account" link. To my surprise, the Web site would not let me cancel my account with the click of a button, instead requiring me to call and giving me a phone number. I thought this was odd and would have expected things to be the other way around. As a computer scientist, I know the process could be automated and made easy for the instructors. Nevertheless, following the instructions, I dialed the number that was written on the Web site.

The customer service representative that I was connected to was, at first, very pleasant. He sounded like he was concerned and wanted to find out the reason why I was resigning. I thought he was genuinely interested in hearing my feedback. But then he quickly started to offer me different options other than cancelling. I was told I could freeze my account at a reduced rate. He also explained that I could encounter difficulties if I cancelled but then decided to reactivate my account. After five or six attempts, the representative realized that I had made up my mind and at this point his tone immediately changed. He was abrupt, terse. He informed me that I still needed to make one last payment for my instructor dues even though the Web site was "statusing" my account as only being valid for three more weeks from that day. So, I told him:

--"Since you sounded like you were interested in hearing feedback, I just wanted to let you know that the account information on the Web site was definitely reporting misleading information on account statuses."

And to my surprise, he replied rather rudely:

-- "You need to contact our technical support for Web site issues."

Here I was, resigning from the company, and he wanted me to contact the technical support department to help them fix their Web site issues? His attitude was rude and uncaring to say the least. I finally realized, however, that I was just talking to a guy whose main job was to find a way to keep me as a monthly paying instructor for as long as possible. In the end, I gave him the instructions to withdraw the last payment they needed on my account and canceled my subscription.

Of course, this representative may have been an exception, and I realize you can't judge an entire company from talking to a single uncaring customer service representative. But the Web site was misleading, leading you to believe you could click in one spot to cancel, when they actually forced you to call in order to allow the company another opportunity to change your mind. And when added up with my experiences with the company and its leadership from the beginning...the hypocrisy and attitude of the customer service rep really summed up the level of experience and support right to the very end.

It opened my eyes to see that any effort by the company to put forth concern and care for customers and employees is a façade in front of the product to make business transactions. I am not naïve - this was not a surprise to me that it occurs - but it did surprise me from company X. I had worked with and served the company for so long, and in that instant I recognized that full other side of that coin for what it was. You see, I realized that for the last six years my passion for the company had been a one way relationship. I presumed that my relationship with them was the same as mine to my students and the instructors I worked with. All of that - the interaction between my peers and students - was genuine and sincere, designed to help each other and be mutually beneficial. But I realized that this is what the company exploits. Every experience I had behind-the-scenes as an agent of the company proved how ruthless this company was right to the very core. And don't think it didn't hurt.

ACT V
WHY I QUIT

16 LACK OF SUPPORT

I remember the launch of the XYZ program and the backlash from other instructors. They had no idea what the program was about, and there were many discussions questioning the value of the program when instructors could learn dance choreography from YouTube, social media, numerous dance videos, DVDs, and more. So many instructors were not supportive and even more would not attend the XYZ sessions, doubting the value. To this date, even after resigning from being an XYZ, I disagree with these feelings. I still see and believe in the program's value! Of course you can learn new dance routines from YouTube and many other means, but there is more to a session than choreography. Even an experienced instructor can network with his or her peers, learning a lot from the other attendees. If you want to advance your career; if you believe in learning, inspiration, and networking; and if you are open to new styles and perspectives, this program provides great value. The lack of systems and tools paralyzes XYZ's, however. What could potentially be a great program is hindered by this lack of tools, and this is evident by the instructors' lack of knowledge as to the benefits of the program which in turn leads to low attendance at sessions. This then yields a significant lack of potential earnings for the XYZ's, who spend countless hours to prepare for his or her sessions. It is a downward spiral, precipitated by the poor foundation, and the results for the XYZ's are unfair.

This is not to say that the tools alone would make every XYZ successful. Of course each XYZ still needs to have the skills and the right mindset to be successful in his or her career. It is important to realize that, even though there is a lack of tools at the time of the writing of this book, a committed XYZ can make many sessions successful, but the work is that much harder. It takes an extreme commitment, including hours of networking on top of hours of preparation on top of hours put into travel to and from sessions on top of the energy and time into conducting the session itself. And in the end, you must be okay in knowing that the monetary reward may not be there.

An XYZ also has to be careful not to use the lack of tools and the controversy between the instructors on the value of the program as excuses. XYZ's can become successful despite the obstacles in their way. And it depends on your definition of success anyway. Success doesn't always mean selling out every session. Attendance numbers are great, but are not always the determination of success. If your heart is in the right place, if you provided the training material in all your sessions, and if you represented the program as it is supposed to be, I believe you are successful. Hopefully that means that eventually your sessions will be full. However, support to make XYZ's successful in their journey is very much needed. I have provided input and suggestions on improvement ideas on numerous occasions after most of my sessions, and I have sent separate emails to the home office and commented on well-watched private XYZ forums for the sake of helping the program and the rest of the XYZ's. I can only hope that eventually help will come.

17 QUANTITY VS QUALITY

I do believe a minimum session requirement is productive. It ensures XYZ's stay active in the program, sharpening their XYZ skills and promoting themselves regularly. However, the current number of required sessions set by the company is overwhelming. It feels like the company wants full-time XYZ's who can focus all their efforts on their sessions year round and this was just not feasible for me and many other XYZ's who signed on with me. I think it is more advantageous to have a program that focuses on quality over quantity. If a session rating is low, the XYZ can be coached to improve, and a more select number of excellent sessions would result. Improvements that focused on quality would better serve and support the program and keep the experienced XYZ's engaged rather than pushing them to the breaking point due to exhaustion, burnout and stress associated in keeping their teaching status.

The fact is that the more sessions an XYZ books, the more money the home office makes. In a best case scenario, increasing the requirements would be a good thing for both the XYZ's *and* the home office. However, the continued lack of support makes this a far more profitable deal for the home office than for the XYZs. XYZ's from smaller or remote areas suffer more due to increased traveling costs to go to areas where more instructors are centralized. And yet, there were never any minimum attendance requirements to coincide with the minimum session requirements to ensure profitable sessions. And the home office was not inclined to push instructors due to the possibility of losing instructors' monthly dues. Those who attend XYZ sessions do so because they either see the value provided, they want to support the XYZ's, and/or they understand the amount of effort that goes into the preparations and promotions of each of these sessions. Some instructors are well aware that the XYZ is under pressure to recover the cost of booking the session.

I have met so many amazing instructors through my sessions and co-sessions with other XYZ's; instructors with big hearts and a love for the program and the people involved with it. But it started to feel unfair to ask for these instructors' continued support while the rest were non-supportive and ignored the fact that the program even existed. After all, there was no requirement for them to participate. And there was definitely no incentive or acknowledgement for the supportive and involved instructors. Even after all the feedback that I personally provided, the company refused to take action or provide any mitigation to ease this situation, and a non-response was the only answer I ever received.

18 PAY OFF

They say to make money, you need to spend money. XYZ's need to invest constantly, keeping up their additional required certifications, keeping the required insurances current, attending conferences, keeping dance and teaching skills relevant, paying for travel, lodging, meals and marketing materials, as well as paying the company their monthly instructor dues just like any other instructor. XYZ's also need to spend countless hours networking, attending other events and listening to new songs that are sent from the home office. They are expected to choreograph to the new songs in future sessions and to create private choreography libraries. The time all this was taking from my family with no real monetary rewards started to feel selfish and became very discouraging. In other words, my "passion" was taking too much time away from my family and was pushing my life out of balance. Coupled with the lack of support, my passion, which had little to no need for monetary return in the first place, started to diminish rapidly as the perception of greed seemed to become the motive for the company.

When I started questioning the value "I" was getting from the XYZ sessions and the value of "my" time and efforts, I felt it was not serving me or the community any longer, especially when I was devoting time to the strict and limiting XYZ sessions when I could be free and guide instructors and students in a more liberating and intellectual way. My time and experience was more valuable and better spent elsewhere than in an XYZ session.

19 GROWING COMPANY, CHANGING ATTITUDES

As the company grew, XYZ operations were delegated to a group of people working at an XYZ specific department. I understand the need may have been there, but the attitude that emerged was "If you do (or don't do) this, your status as an XYZ will be removed permanently." Or "Since you did this, you will no longer be eligible for this." Such were the types of communications we received from this new department - threats of harsh consequences that were a cross between a dictatorship and kindergarten-management style. There are ways to have rules and requirements (and a need for them, to be sure) while still treating XYZ's as responsible adults and recognizing them for the overwhelming efforts and countless hours put forth towards the massive growth of the entire program. And when XYZ's have questions or suggestions, the company needs to follow them up with an appropriate response.

20 DOUBLE STANDARD

Maybe this is controversial to some, but I need to be honest and bring you my full perspective, even if this is just my personal value statement. To be silent would not do you or me any justice. As you were reading throughout my early career experiences, I touched on a few incidents that deep down I knew were wrong but ignored them anyway. Maybe I ignored the warning signs because I was so excited about the opportunities. Maybe I was too blind because of my passion. Maybe I was too forgiving because I thought I was helping my students and instructors along the way. Maybe I was too naïve because the fitness industry was new to me, and I was making my own mistakes. It probably doesn't matter the reason(s) why, but there were definitely red flags I should have paid attention to that pointed to unfair and double standards that were very real.

YouTube stars were hired by the company when other instructors were being told that YouTube was forbidden and not to post videos. (I have no problem with anybody trying to use the tools available today to help promote and advance their career, but I also understand the legal requirements and protecting the brand of a company, legality of the songs, etc. In other words, as a company owner, I wouldn't want my company represented poorly on a YouTube video so I, too, would probably restrict the usage of the platform. But the rule would also apply the other way around, meaning you shouldn't be rewarded by the same company for then breaking those rules, even if the work was considered a good representation.)

Another double standard was that I wrote an e-book earlier on that was intended to be of value for other instructors in helping promote their fitness events. When company X found out, however, it was banned because of a reference to the company name. At the same time, there were other books on the market also using the company name (referenced many times) that were not banned. I ended up changing the name and references throughout the book so I could publish my book again, but it is another example of a double standard with no explanation or communication as to why others' works were permissible when mine was not.

There were a lot of requirements for and micro-management of the trainings and sessions for the XYZ's, but very few requirements were put on the instructors other than attending that first day of training and paying their monthly dues. While educators were (and still are) paying the same dues for the company as all the rest of the instructors, the requirements appeared to make educators less important and more disposable since there are thousands of other instructors who desired the same job and the millions of monthly dues are much more difficult to disregard than a few hundred monthly dues coming from the educators.

All the things we were forbidden to do as XYZ's, such as marketing our sessions on social media, were allowed when it came to marketing and advertising the events that were organized by the company. In those instances, XYZ's were specifically *instructed* to market these events on social media - by the very same company! I do believe in supporting a company for which I work, but not when it comes to obvious double standards and hypocrisy.

After dealing with no support from the home office, along with the double standards, unprofessional and unreasonable treatment towards XYZ's, dealing with frantic schedules and changing requirements benefiting only the front office, I started to question the integrity of the company, and my attitude became resentful. I started to feel "exploited" with little return or company recognition of the investment of my time and efforts. I started to question if I was even a good fit for this position and the company any longer.

21 "SELFISH" REASONS

As I mentioned earlier, in 2013 we dealt with a major life event, moving from the West Coast to the East Coast. Going through the emotions and challenges of the move and adjusting to a new environment, I asked myself three key questions:

Question #1: Knowing what I knew at the time, three years ago, would I still apply for this position? The answer was absolutely "yes." The three years were an amazing growth experience for me, and I am so grateful for all the friendships and bonds I made with instructors and students throughout my classes and XYZ sessions. They are priceless relationships, and I met so many amazing people during the journey. But then I had to ask the next two questions:

Question #2: Knowing what I know *now*, including the years of financial, emotional and physical investment I have made and despite how things might be a year from now, would I still apply for this position?

Question #3: If I had only six months to live, would I still be doing this job and does this job and company line up with my true values and where I want to be 5-10 years from now?

I think you know the answers I had to the last two questions.

22 CONCLUSION

You never know when life is going to throw something new and challenging at you. Sometimes a major life event (hopefully not health-related), needs to happen for you to open your eyes and see things from a different angle. Sometimes you need to remove yourself from a situation and look at it as if your friend was in your shoes. What would you advise your friend to do? Today I feel extremely lucky and fortunate to be able to live my life with an abundance of support from my family and friends, and I feel extremely blessed because I am able to work hard and reap the rewards for the work I do. I lead a very comfortable life, and I pray every day that it continues.

I am also grateful for the opportunity I had being an XYZ because the journey was an amazing learning experience. Even the lack of tools and support from the company brought some good results – it forced me to create and implement tools for myself, taught me how to sell to others, and showed me how to start a business on my own.

There are so many XYZ's who are extremely talented and who display such passion for what they do, and I will continue to support every one of them in their journeys. I hope that my experience helps them support their case when it is their turn to ask for the things that I did. The truth is, I would still be an XYZ if things had been different.

Today, I am living my life by design, exercising and including fitness in my life on my own terms. I am spending more quality time with my family and have many new and exciting projects that I focus on. I am happier, have more energy, and live a less frantic and stress-free life which I know is better for my health, even when considering all of the strenuous cardio sessions I used to have! I am pursuing leadership and teaching opportunities in different ways. I am blessed to recognize that with today's technology, I can contribute to people's lives "virtually" and not just in person. I know that people are smiling back at me; I can feel it even if I don't see it. My friends and followers are still there, supporting me and cheering me on. Today, I am lucky to be able to write this book and have the time to reflect on my experience. I am grateful for the life change it took for me to be able to stop, think, and do a "reality check." Sometimes we need to get back in line with our true values through a life self-assessment. I hope that you, in reading this book, will find inspiration, focus, and self-help in your own journey through life.

ABOUT THE AUTHOR

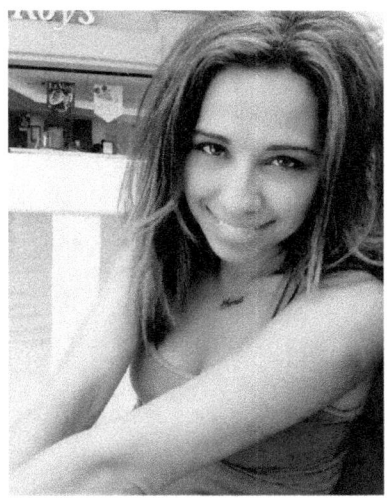

Arzu Gosney was born in Istanbul, Turkiye (Turkey). She grew up in Turkey and came to America in 1999 to pursue a Masters degree in Computer Science. After completing her masters and PhD. in Computer Science at Washington State University, she stayed on to teach Computer Science courses. Her practical work experience consists of Just in Time inventory management for an automotive company in Turkey; IT Developer; and IT Manager at National Department of Energy Laboratory in the United States of America. Her doctoral research is in Adaptive Scientific Workflows in High Performance Computing. Arzu has a passion for fitness and has been a fitness instructor for six years. She loves teaching, learning and making a difference in other's career, health, and lives.

CONNECT WITH ARZU

Blog: https://arzugosney.com
Facebook: https://facebook.com/arzugosneypage
Twitter: https://twitter.com/arzugosney
Amazon Author Central Site (includes all the links to Arzu's books): http://www.amazon.com/Arzu-Gosney/e/B00GQZ6TDU/

ONE LAST THING

Thanks for reading! If you enjoyed this book or found it useful or inspirational I would be grateful if you would post a short review. Your support really does make a difference, and I read all the reviews personally so I can get your feedback and make this book even better.

Thank you again for your support!